Corinne Bähler

Non-perforating abomasal lesions in veal calves

Corinne Bähler

Non-perforating abomasal lesions in veal calves

Effects of the two production programs 'Naturafarm' and 'conventional' on the prevalence of non-perforating abomasal lesions

Südwestdeutscher Verlag für Hochschulschriften

Impressum/Imprint (nur für Deutschland/ only for Germany)
Bibliografische Information der Deutschen Nationalbibliothek: Die Deutsche Nationalbibliothek verzeichnet diese Publikation in der Deutschen Nationalbibliografie; detaillierte bibliografische Daten sind im Internet über http://dnb.d-nb.de abrufbar.

Alle in diesem Buch genannten Marken und Produktnamen unterliegen warenzeichen-, marken- oder patentrechtlichem Schutz bzw. sind Warenzeichen oder eingetragene Warenzeichen der jeweiligen Inhaber. Die Wiedergabe von Marken, Produktnamen, Gebrauchsnamen, Handelsnamen, Warenbezeichnungen u.s.w. in diesem Werk berechtigt auch ohne besondere Kennzeichnung nicht zu der Annahme, dass solche Namen im Sinne der Warenzeichen- und Markenschutzgesetzgebung als frei zu betrachten wären und daher von jedermann benutzt werden dürften.

Verlag: Südwestdeutscher Verlag für Hochschulschriften Aktiengesellschaft & Co. KG
Dudweiler Landstr. 99, 66123 Saarbrücken, Deutschland
Telefon +49 681 37 20 271-1, Telefax +49 681 37 20 271-0
Email: info@svh-verlag.de
Zugl.: Bern, Vetsuisse-Fakultät, Diss., 2008

Herstellung in Deutschland:
Schaltungsdienst Lange o.H.G., Berlin
Books on Demand GmbH, Norderstedt
Reha GmbH, Saarbrücken
Amazon Distribution GmbH, Leipzig
ISBN: 978-3-8381-1243-5

Imprint (only for USA, GB)
Bibliographic information published by the Deutsche Nationalbibliothek: The Deutsche Nationalbibliothek lists this publication in the Deutsche Nationalbibliografie; detailed bibliographic data are available in the Internet at http://dnb.d-nb.de.

Any brand names and product names mentioned in this book are subject to trademark, brand or patent protection and are trademarks or registered trademarks of their respective holders. The use of brand names, product names, common names, trade names, product descriptions etc. even without a particular marking in this works is in no way to be construed to mean that such names may be regarded as unrestricted in respect of trademark and brand protection legislation and could thus be used by anyone.

Publisher: Südwestdeutscher Verlag für Hochschulschriften Aktiengesellschaft & Co. KG
Dudweiler Landstr. 99, 66123 Saarbrücken, Germany
Phone +49 681 37 20 271-1, Fax +49 681 37 20 271-0
Email: info@svh-verlag.de

Printed in the U.S.A.
Printed in the U.K. by (see last page)
ISBN: 978-3-8381-1243-5

Copyright © 2010 by the author and Südwestdeutscher Verlag für Hochschulschriften Aktiengesellschaft & Co. KG and licensors
All rights reserved. Saarbrücken 2010

Table of contents

1. Introduction 1
2. Material and Methods
   2.1. Sample collection 4
   2.2. Pathological examination 5
   2.3. Data on farm management, individual animals
        and carcass parameters.. 7
   2.4. Statistics 9
3. Results
   3.1. Data on farm management, individual animals
        and carcass parameters 11
   3.2. Prevalence and types of abomasal lesions.................... 17
   3.3. Risk factor analysis for abomasal lesions in the fundic part.......... 28
   3.4. Risk factor analysis for abomasal lesions in the pyloric part 30
4. Discussion 32
5. Acknowledgements 38
6. References... 39

Effects of the two production programs 'Naturafarm' and 'conventional' on the prevalence of non-perforating abomasal lesions in Swiss veal calves at slaughter

1. Introduction

In order to meet consumers expectations with respect to meat color, calves are fattened with milk and milk by-products beyond the age at which feeding of roughage would be required from a physiological point of view. This situation has long been suspected to contribute to the development of a number of digestive tract disorders including various abomasal lesions. Non-perforating lesions include any defects of the abomasal lining leaving the serosa unpunctered. The reported overall prevalence of non-perforating abomasal lesions in veal calves at slaughter varies from 67% to 95% (Wiepkema et al., 1987; Welchman and Baust, 1987; Groth and Berner, 1971). Non-perforating lesions may cause economic losses by decreasing feed conversion efficiency and predisposing calves to perforating lesions (Bähler, 2007). Non-perforating lesions are susceptible to develop into perforating ulcers involving chronic bleeding and septic peritonitis. Abomasal ulceration is the main cause of death of veal calves in Italy (Cagalli et al., 1995). In Switzerland, perforating abomasal ulcers account for 25% of fatal outcome in veal calves between 3 and 16 weeks of age (Bähler, 2007). The etiopathogenesis of abomasal lesions in veal calves has not been completely elucidated, but it is generally accepted that the disease is related to multiple factors. Roughage with a high fiber content (Morisse et al., 2000; Wensing et *al.*, 1986), large volumes of individual feeding rations combined with a low feeding frequency (Ahmed *et al.*, 2002; Navetat, 1987), and low luminal pH in the abomasum (Constable *et al.*, 2005) all have been suspected to contribute to the development of abomasal lesions. In addition, acute and chronic stress is considered to cause imbalances between aggressive and defensive mechanisms, impairing the integrity of the abomasal mucosa (Dirksen *et al.*, 1997; Geishauser, 1989; Singh *et al.*, 1967). In those studies in which localization of the lesions was taken into account, the authors hypothesized that dissimilar factors may produce the lesions in the fundic part and the pyloric part, respectively (Gesper and Dirksen, 1988; Hemmingsen, 1966; Jelinski *et al.*, 1996; Krauser, 1987; Lensink *et al.*, 2000). In the abomasal fundus, secretion of acid and mucus is analogous to the stomach of human beings and other monogastric species such as rats and mice, where several physical and psychological factors have been alleged to produce mucosal lesions (Katagiri *et al.*, 2005; Meddings and Swain, 2000; Santos *et al.*, 2001; Saunders *et al.*, 1997). Lesions in the pyloric part were attributed to the repeated intake of high volumes of milk or milk replacer (Bokkers and Koene, 2001; Veissier *et al.*, 2001). In a considerable number of previous investigations on abomasal lesions in calves, the localization of the abomasal lesions, unfortunately, was not considered.

'*Conventional*' veal production settings in Switzerland conform to the minimal standards of animal welfare as based on the Swiss animal welfare legislation (Tierschutzgesetz 1978). There is an increasing demand by Swiss consumers for 'animal-friendly' production which meets standards exceeding current animal welfare regulations. Consequently, the veal production program *'Naturafarm'* (Coop, 2004) was created four years ago by Coop, the country's second-largest retailer. Enhanced animal welfare requirements include minimizing transportation time to a maximum of 6 hours, allocation of the calves to the fattening unit at a minimum age of 21 days, low stocking density (at least 3.5 m^2 per calf), permanent free access to an outdoor pen and to fresh water, and feeding roughage ad libitum. These measures were expected to reduce stress and enhance the overall health status of the calves.

The objective of our study was to evaluate the overall prevalence and severity of pyloric and/or fundic abomasal lesions in Swiss veal calves at slaughter and to compare the frequency of abomasal lesions between *'Naturafarm'*-calves and calves kept under minimal standards of the Swiss animal welfare legislation (group *'conventional'*). In order to identify individual risk factors for the development of abomasal lesions, we comprehensively analyzed management, housing and feeding factors.

2. Material and Methods

2.1. Sample collection

All samples were collected in one large abattoir where 20% of the Swiss veal calves are slaughtered. Over a period of 6 months (June 2006 to December 2006), abomasa of 125 calves were randomly selected. As a rule, calves were slaughtered on one or two days per week and were delivered from 4 a.m. on. *'Naturafarm'*- and *'conventional'*-calves were kept separate for transport as well as in the waiting area of the slaughterhouse. Calves from different production settings entered the slaughtering area randomly. Each time, about ten abomasa of each production group were collected within a maximum of two hours after delivery of the calves to the slaughterhouse. Abomasa were labeled for identification. After collection, every abomasum was packed in a plastic box which was kept in a cold storage room at the slaughterhouse (18°C). For the one-hour-transport to the Veterinary School of Bern, the air-conditioning system of the car was adjusted to 18°C, prior to loading the plastic box with the abomasa. Upon arrival, abomasa were immediately opened along the great curvature and rinsed for macroscopic examination. Individual ear tags allowed identification of calves and their provenance (*'Naturafarm'* or *'conventional'*) through the Swiss national farm and animal movement database. The examiner had no clue as to the origin of the abomasa.

2.2. Pathological examination

Within at most four hours after collecting the material, abomasa were inspected macroscopically at the Vetsuisse Faculty of Berne. Location of any macroscopic lesion was specifically recorded for the fundic and the pyloric regions. Lesions on the torus were ranked among pyloric lesions. The torus is a bulge that rises from the small curvature into the pyloric lumen (Dyce et al., 1991). Lesions were classified according to the categorization of Braun et al. (1991) and Wiepkema et al. (1987) with minor adaptations. Lesions of Type 1: Superficial erosions with minimal mucosal defects and mucosal discolorations. Type 2: Deeper erosions, the center of the lesions clearly depressed. Type 3: Craters with a superficial coating, apparent loss of tissue, central depression. Type 4: Deep craters, the center of the lesion being depressed and hemorrhagic. Disputable lesions of Type 1 were processed for histological assessment. According to Wiepkema et al. (1987), Type 1 was assumed to be the most benign lesion, whereas Type 4 was considered to be the most serious lesion. Where appropriate, specific staining methods were performed according to Prophet et al. (1994). In order to demonstrate the presence of Iron, Perls Iron Stain was used. Slides were placed in freshly mixed hydrochloric acid-potassium ferrocyanide for 30 minutes (final concentration: 10% hydrochloric acid, 5% potassium ferrocyanide). Sections were rinsed in distilled water and counterstained with nuclear fast red solution for 5 minutes. Degradation of hemoglobin as an indicator of chronic bleeding was visualized by means of the periodic acid Schiff procedure. This involved the oxidation of deparaffinized sections in 0.5% periodic acid solution for 5 minutes. After rinsing the slides in distilled water, sections were placed in Coleman's Schiff reagent (0.5% basic fuchsin and 1% potassium metabisulfite) for 15 minutes. After thorough rinsing in tap water, counterstaining was carried out with Mayer's hematoxylin solution for 15 minutes. Presence of fungi was substantiated using Grocott's methenamine silver nitrate method. Sections were oxidized in fresh 4% chromic acid solution for 1 hour. A brief rinse in tap water was followed by a 1 minute exposure to 1% sodium bisulfate solution. After a thorough rinse with tap and distilled water, sections were incubated in methenamine-silver nitrate solution (final concentration: 0.125% silver nitrate and 1.5% methenamine) at 59^0C for 1 hour. Subsequent to another thorough rinse in distilled water, sections were toned in 0.1% gold chloride solution for 4 minutes. Rinsed slides were then placed in 5% sodium thiosulfate solution for 4 minutes and washed again. Counterstaining implicated exposure to 0.03% light green solution for 40 seconds.

2.3. Data on farm management, individual animals and carcass parameters

A structured questionnaire was used in order to survey the owners about farm management parameters. A full length version of the questionnaire in German may be requested from the corresponding author, a summary is provided in Table 1. Questions addressed and information collected included the type of farm, origin of the calves, production program, animal flow system, number of fattening groups and group size, type of barn, cleaning intensity of the barn, ventilation system and whether calves had outdoor access. Additional questions were about the feeding frequency, feeding technique, and whether calves had permanent access to fresh water and/or hay (dried grass; averaged constituents per kg dry matter: organic matter 906 g, crude fibre 220 g, crude protein 137 g (RAP, 1999)), and on feed type. Milk by-products (Amobolac and Protofit) originated from cheese dairies, and proteins, fructose and fat were added by homogenization or with emulgators. Supplementary powder (Gefumilk and Sprayfit) was produced by processing milk by-products in a spray tower, and by adding proteins, fructose, fat, minerals and vitamins. The liquid milk by-products and the supplementary powders were produced under low heat.

Data collected by questionnaire were used for a risk factor analysis with the aim to identify farm management practices and animal characteristics which are associated with an increased risk of abomasal lesions at slaughter. Data about the calves (sex, age at slaughter, breed) were obtained from the Swiss national farm and animal movement database and carcass data (quality and color) were registered and stored electronically by the slaughterhouse system. Carcass quality was scored according to the Swiss standard in five categories (C,H,T,A,X), whereas C represents the highest and X the lowest quality. For risk factor analysis, the categories C and H were subsumed to high quality, T to medium quality, A and X to low quality. Carcass color was also scored in three categories (white, pink, red) according to Swiss standards.

2.4. Statistics

All analyses were performed using the NCSS 97 System for Windows version XP (NCSS 97, Kaysville, Utah). Abomasa were classified according to the macroscopical presence or absence of lesions in the fundic and pyloric (including torus) part, respectively. Risk factors for lesions in both anatomical regions were analyzed separately, because their etiology was suspected to be different. Therefore, the prevalence of these different lesions might depend on different risk factors. Two separate multivariate regression models were analyzed with presence of fundic and pyloric lesions as the dependent variable, respectively. In a first step, factors were screened for significant association with the dependent variable with univariable logistic regression. Variables associated with the presence of abomasal lesions ($p < 0.2$) were entered into a multivariate logistic regression model. With a stepwise backward variable selection procedure, only variables significant at $p < 0.05$ were retained in the model. In case of highly correlated variables, the biologically more-plausible variable was left in the model. For example, the feeding frequency was kept in the model instead of the type of barn, because a causal relationship between abomasal lesions and feeding frequency seemed more plausible than with the type of barn. After deletion of a non-significant variable, we checked whether the model log likelihood changed significantly, and whether the regression coefficients of the remaining variables changed by > 25%. If either of these was the case, that non-significant variable was retained in the model. Interactions between significant variables were only analyzed if they were biologically meaningful. Odds ratios, 95% confidence intervals of the odds ratio, and Wald's p-value were used to describe the results of the logistic regression models.

3. Results

3.1. Data on farm management, individual animals and carcass parameters

125 abomasa were collected on a total of six slaughtering days. Sixty-four calves originated from 14 'Naturafarm' farms and 61 calves from 32 'conventional' farms. Complete farm management data were available for all samples. Characteristics of the farms as obtained by the questionnaire are summarized and categorized in Table 1. On most farms of both production programs, the primary income was generated from milk production. The calves were mainly purchased on markets, pre-existing cow or pig barns had been reconstructed for veal production, barns were manually ventilated by windows, and calves were fed *ad libitum* by an automatic feeding system. Differences between 'Naturafarm'- and 'conventional'-farms concerned the animal flow system, the cleaning intensity of the barn, the access to an outside pen, the number of fattening groups per farm, group size, the availability of water and hay, and the feed type. On most of the 'Naturafarm'-farms, calves were fed a milk by-product (Amobolac or Protofit) plus supplementary powder (Gefumilk or Sprayfit), and on most 'conventional' farms, calves were fed whole milk plus supplementary powder (Meliormilk). Contents of liquid milk-products and powders are compiled in Table 2. The ingredients of the liquid milk by-product Amobolac were skim milk, whey, fat, fructose, and milk protein, whereas the other milk by-product Protofit was made up of buttermilk, skim milk, whey, fat, fructose, wheat starch, milk

protein, and emulgators. The mean age at slaughter was 148 days (range 119 to 202 days) for *'Naturafarm'* calves and 155 days (range from 115 to 220 days) for calves raised in *'conventional'* settings. The mean carcass weight of the *'Naturafarm'* calves was 123 kg (range from 96 to 150 kg) and that of *'conventional'* calves was 126 kg (range from 110 to 149 kg). Animals' data (sex and breed) and carcass data (quality and color) are summarized in Table 3. In both production programs, most animals were male, of dairy breeds, and their carcasses were of medium quality (T). With respect to carcass color, most of the *'Naturafarm'* calves were pink, whereas most *'conventional'* calves had a white carcass color.

Table 1.
Descriptive data obtained by questionnaire about the veal farms participating in the study, illustrated according to the production programs 'Naturafarm' and 'conventional'

Factor	Number of 'Naturafarm' farms (n=14)	In %	Number of 'conventional' farms (n=32)	In %
Main income by				
Veal production	1	7	0	0
Dairy cows	9	65	26	81
Pig production	2	14	0	0
Agriculture	1	7	0	0
Other branches	1	7	6	19
Purchase				
Mainly calves from the own farm	5	36	15	47
Mainly purchase on market	9	64	17	53
Animal flow system				
Continuously	4	29	23	72
All-in-all-out	10	71	9	28
Type of building				
Reconstruction of an existing barn	12	86	27	84
New barn	2	14	5	16
Ventilation technique				
Open fronted barn	0	0	1	3
Manual ventilation by windows	8	57	20	63
Artificial (Ventilator)	6	43	11	34
Cleaning intensity (per fattening period)				
More than once	5	36	20	63
Once	8	57	10	31
Less than once	1	7	2	6
Permanent outdoor access				
Yes	14	100	5	16
No	0	0	27	84
Number of fattening groups per farm				
One	8	58	12	38
Two	3	21	16	50
Three	3	21	4	12

Factor	Number of 'Naturafarm' farms (n=14)	In %	Number of 'conventional' farms (n=32)	In %
Group size				
1-10	1	7	17	53
11-20	4	29	8	25
21-30	1	7	4	13
31-40	7	50	2	6
>40	1	7	1	3
Feeding frequency				
Twice daily	0	0	13	41
Ad libitum	14	100	19	59
Feeding technique				
By bucket with artificial teat	0	0	6	19
By bucket without artificial teat	0	0	7	22
By automatic system	14	100	19	59
Feed type				
Whole milk plus Meliormilk	5	36	27	84
Amobolac plus Gefumilk	4	28	1	3
Protofit plus Sprayfit	5	36	4	13
Free access to fresh water				
Yes	14	100	13	41
No	0	0	19	59
Free access to hay				
Yes	14	100	9	28
No	0	0	23	72

Table 2.
Contents of milk, liquid milk by-products and supplementary powders fed to veal calves of the production groups 'Naturafarm' and 'conventional'

Liquid product	Water in %	Crude protein g / kg DM*	Crude fat g / kg DM	Crude ash g / kg DM	pH	Vegetal ingredients in %
Whole milk	87.0	33	40	7	6.8	--
Amobolac	67	64--67	71-74	20	6.0-6.2	--
Protofit	70-71	54-57	56-59	12-15	5.6-6.0	--
Supplementary powder						
Meliormilk	--	270	160	--	--	4%
Gefumilk	--	270	120	--	--	< 2%
Sprayfit	--	320	120	--	--	No declaration

Table 3.

Sex, breed and carcass data of the veal calves, illustrated according to the production programs 'Naturafarm' and 'conventional'

Factor	'Naturafarm' calves (n=64)	In %	'conventional' calves (n=61)	In %
Sex				
Male	40	63	51	84
Female	24	37	10	16
Breed				
Dairy breeds	45	70	44	72
Cross breeds	14	22	16	26
Other breeds	5	8	1	2
Carcass quality				
High quality (C, H)	17	27	10	16
Medium quality (T)	42	65	50	82
Low quality (A. X)	5	8	1	2
Carcass color				
White	16	25	46	75
Pink	35	55	15	25
Red	13	20	0	0

3.2. Prevalence and types of abomasal lesions

As illustrated in Fig. 1, one (1.6%) and 8 (13.1%) abomasa of the groups 'Naturafarm' and 'conventional', respectively, showed lesions only in the fundic part (significant difference, p = 0.03). Fourty-nine (76.6%) and 43 (70.5%) of the abomasa of the groups 'Naturafarm' and 'conventional', respectively, had lesions only in the pyloric part (difference not significant, p = 0.44). Four (6.3%) and 6 (9.8%) abomasa of the groups 'Naturafarm' and 'conventional', respectively, showed lesions in the fundic and pyloric part (difference not significant, p = 0.46). For univariable logistic regression, abomasa were classified according to the presence or absence of lesions, taking into account the anatomical regions of the fundic and pyloric part. Abomasa with lesions in both anatomical regions were classified as presence of lesions in both regression models. There was a significant difference in the frequency of fundic lesions between the two groups: animals raised in a 'conventional' production setting had a significantly higher prevalence of lesions in the fundic part (p = 0.024, odds ratio (OR) = 3.5, confidence interval (CI) = 0.17 – 2.35), whereas there was no significant difference (p = 0.44, OR = 0.73, CI = - 1.11 – 0.40) in the frequency of abomasal lesions in the pyloric region between the groups 'Naturafarm' and 'conventional'.

The distribution of abomasal lesions in the fundic and pyloric part of 'Naturafarm' and 'conventional' calves are presented in Figs. 2 and 3, respectively. Lesions of Type 1 (Fig. A) were present in 4 (6.3%) and 10

(16.4%) abomasa of the groups *'Naturafarm'* and *'conventional'*, respectively, in the fundic area, and 16 (25%) and 7 (11.5%), respectively, in the pyloric area. Lesion of Type 2 (Fig. B) was diagnosed in only one abomasum (1.6%) of the group *'conventional'* in the pyloric part. Lesions of Type 3 (Fig. C) were present in one (1.6%) and 3 (4.9%) abomasa of the groups *'Naturafarm'* and *'conventional'*, respectively, in the fundic part, and 32 (50%) and 35 (57.4%), respectively, in the pyloric part. Lesions of Type 4 (Fig. D) were diagnosed only in the fundic part of one abomasum (1.6%) of the *'conventional'* group and in the pyloric part of one abomasum (1.6%) of the *'Naturafarm'* group. Whenever classification as Type 1 was doubtful, samples were assessed histologically. When neutrophils, lymphocytes, macrophages, and necrosis of the mucosa were present (Figs. E and F), lesions were categorized as Type 1. In cases of no inflammatory infiltration, abomasa were classified as "no lesions".

Fig. 1. Distribution of macroscopic abomasal lesions of 'Naturafarm' and 'conventional' veal calves considering the anatomical regions fundus and pylorus

* Frequency of lesions of corresponding location marked with asterisk (*) are significantly different ($p < 0.05$)

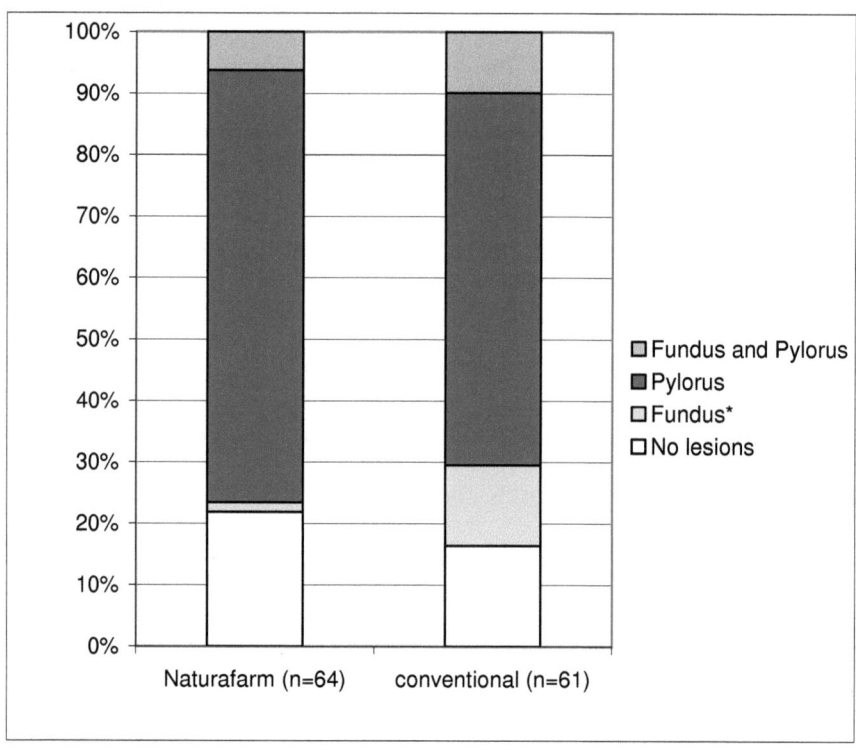

Fig. 2. Frequency of types of macroscopic abomasal lesions (Type 1 to 4) in the fundic part of 'Naturafarm' and 'conventional' veal calves at slaughter

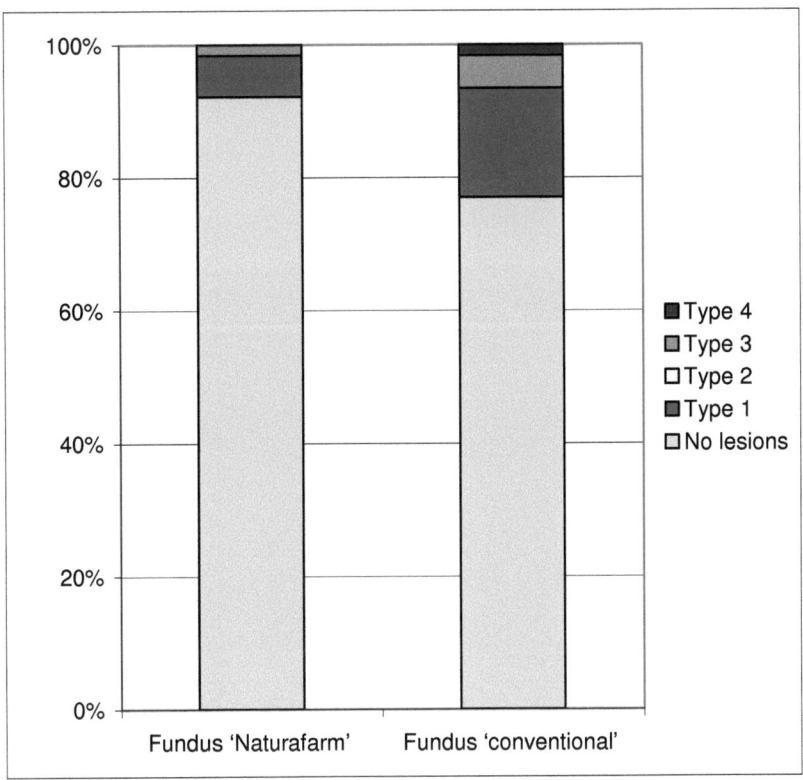

Fig. 3. Frequency of types of macroscopic abomasal lesions (Type 1 to 4) in the pyloric part of *'Naturafarm'* and *'conventional'* veal calves at slaughter

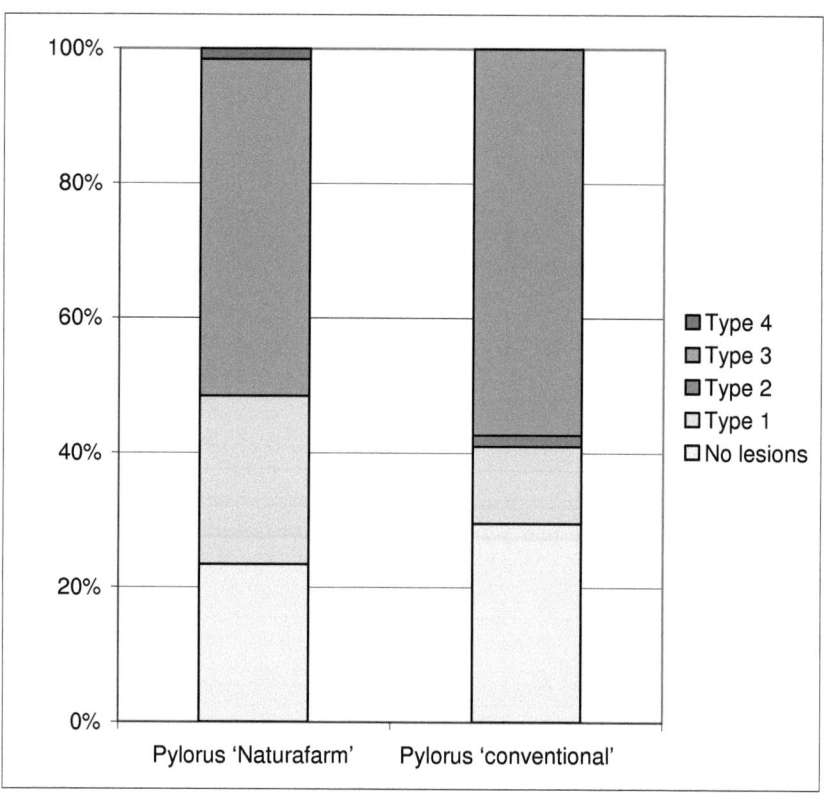

Fig. A. Superficial erosions of the mucosa and sharply demarcated reddish and brownish discolorations (Type 1) in the pyloric mucosa of a *'Naturafarm'* veal calf at slaughter

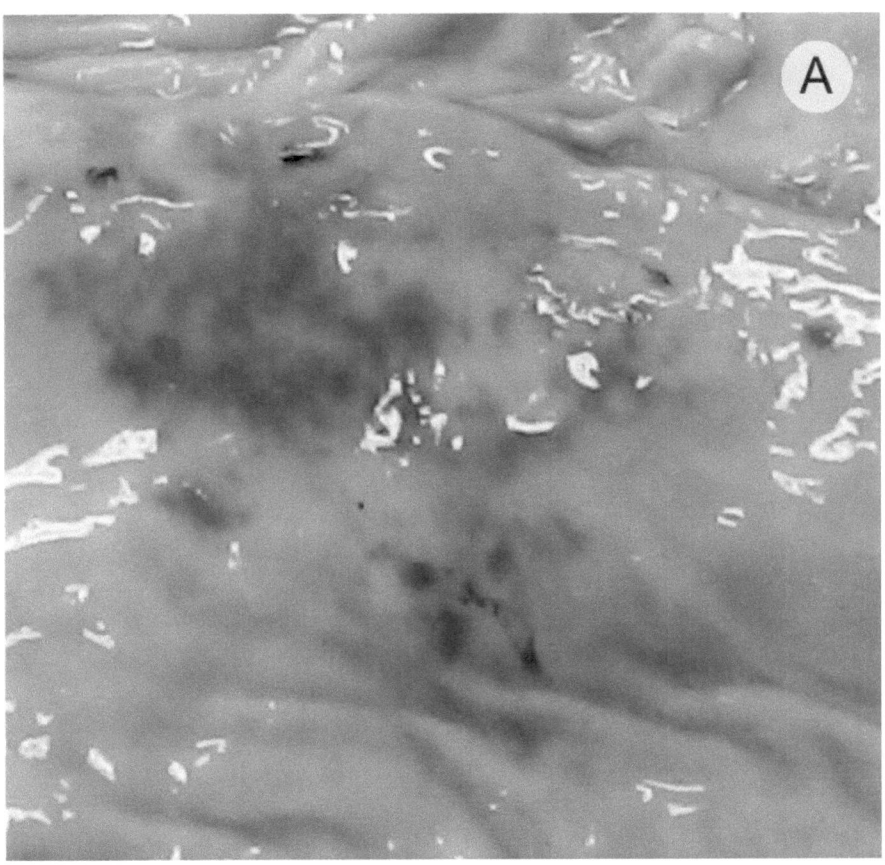

Fig. B. Deeper erosion of the mucosa with a clearly depressed center and reddish discoloration (Type 2) in the pyloric mucosa of a *conventional* veal calf at slaughter

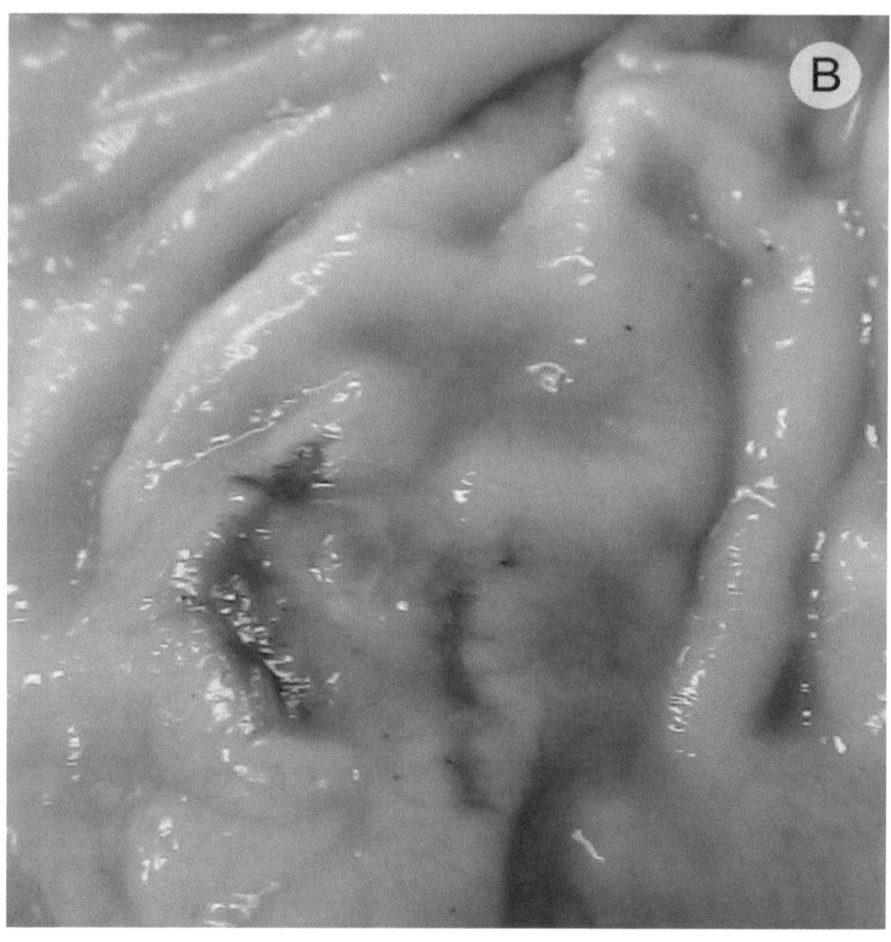

Fig. C. Crater with superficial coating, apparent loss of tissue, and a depressed center of the lesion (Type 3) in the pyloric mucosa of a *'conventional'* veal calf at slaughter

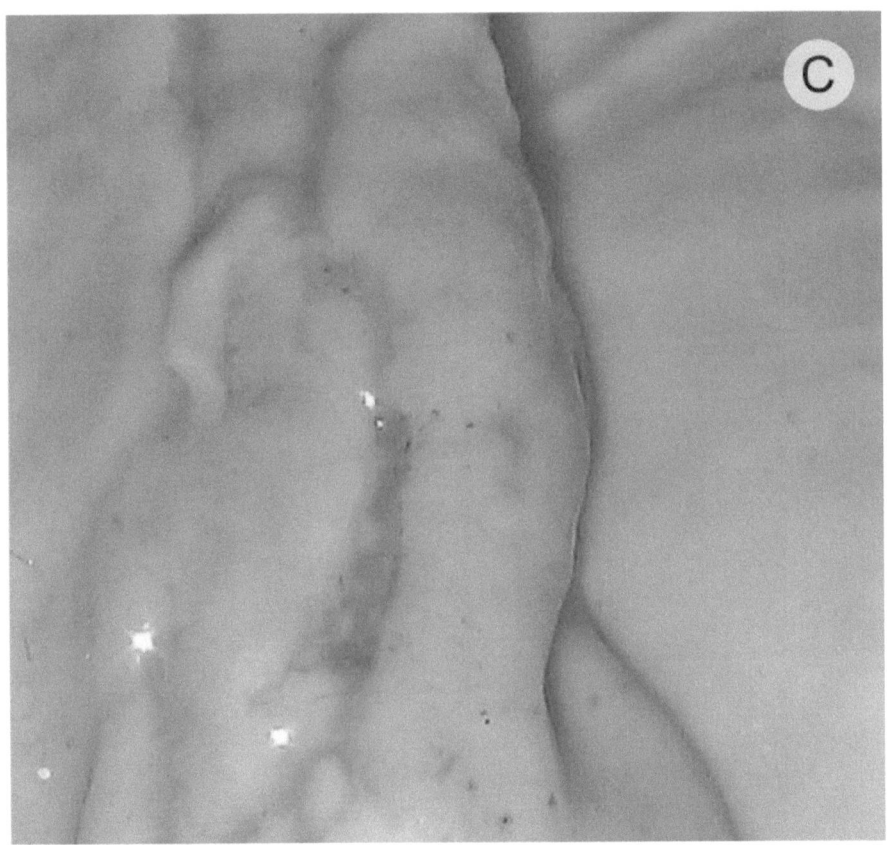

Fig. D. Deep crater, the center of the lesion depressed and hemorrhagic (Type 4) in the pyloric mucosa of a *'Naturafarm'* veal calf at slaughter

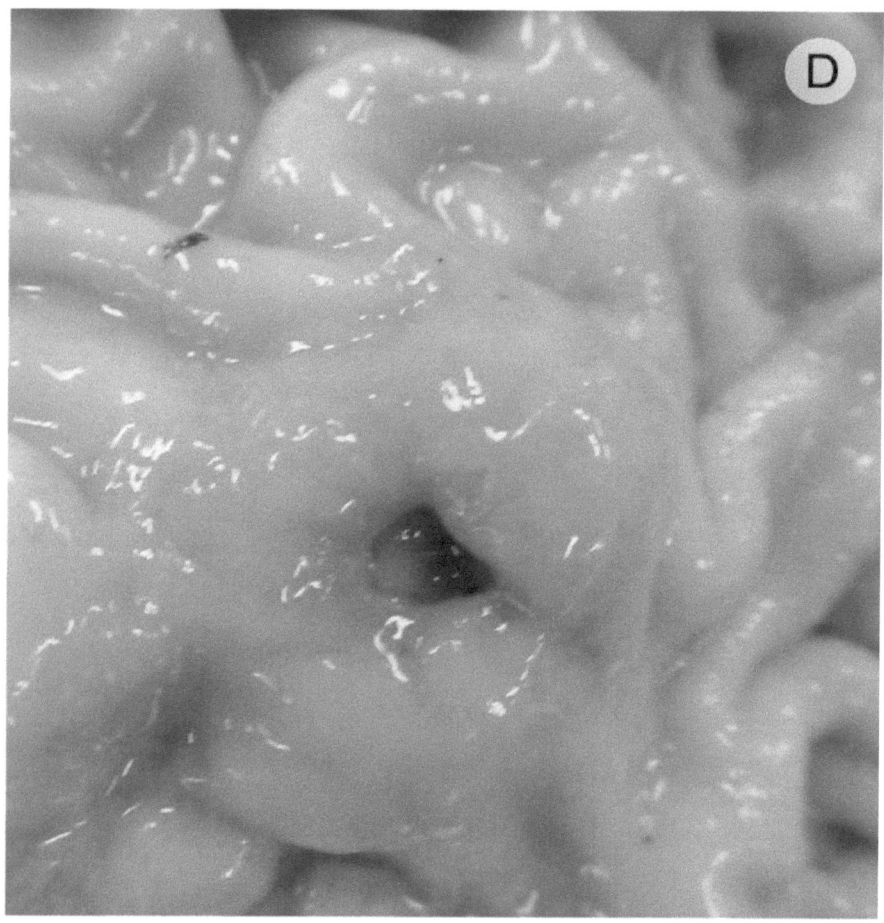

Fig. E. Histological image of Fig. A (Type 1), representing necrosis of the mucosa. 1) Abomasal lumen; 2) Gastric epithelium; 3) Propria with pyloric glands; 4) Necrotic area; Haematoxilin-Eosin staining; original magnification is 50x

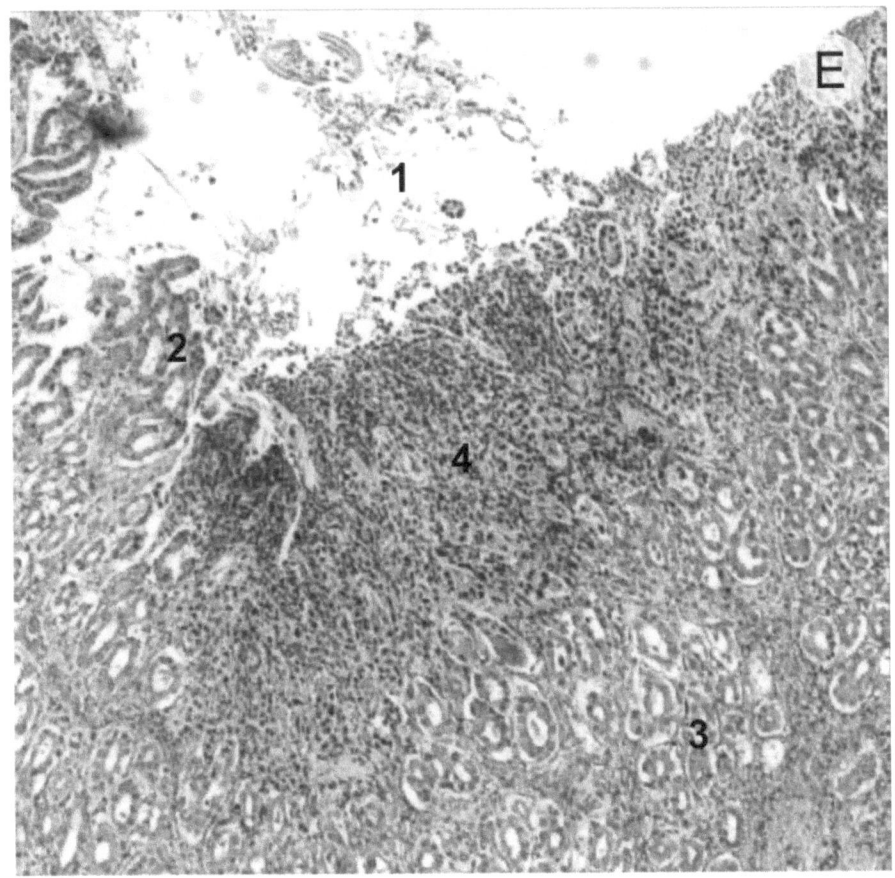

Fig. F. Inset of Fig. E, representing strong infiltration of the propria by neutrophils and macrophages. 1) Pyloric glands; 2) Neutrophils; 3) Macrophages; Haematoxilin-Eosin staining, original magnification is 200x

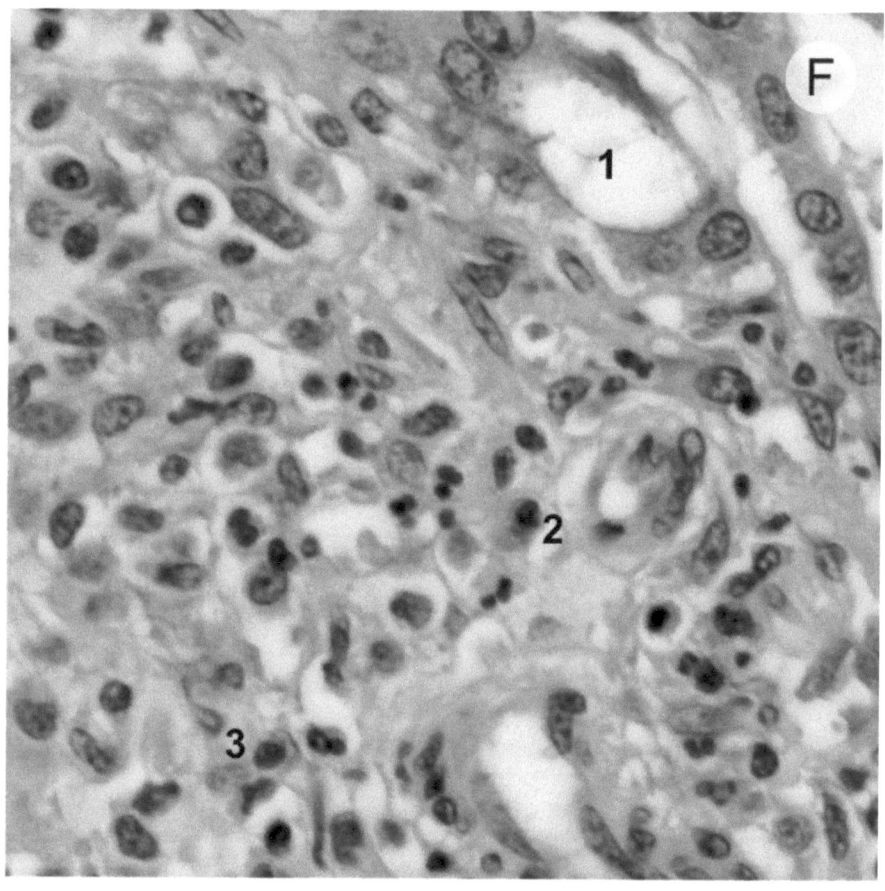

3.3. Risk factor analysis for abomasal lesions in the fundic part

Factors from almost all categories including management, housing, feeding, and carcass data correlated with lesions in the fundic part of the abomasum when tested with univariable logistic regression. As illustrated in Table 4, the number of fattening groups per farm and the group size, the type of building, the feeding frequency and the type of feed, the access to water, and finally the age at slaughter and the carcass quality were weakly associated with abomasal lesions in the fundic part ($0.05 < y < 0.2$). A high correlation ($p < 0.05$) with an increased risk for fundic lesions was observed for the production type, for the availability of an outside pen, feeding by bucket with an artificial teat, and free access to hay. In multivariate logistic regression analysis, the type of feed, the feeding technique, and the production type were the risk factors being significantly associated with abomasal lesions in the fundic part (Table 5).

Table 5.
Factors highly associated (p < 0.05) with the risk for occurrence of macroscopic abomasal lesions in the fundic part of veal calves at slaughter (multivariate logistic regression)

Factor	Reference	Odds ratio	95% Confidence interval	Wald's p-value (p)
Bucket with artificial teat	Automatic feeding system	12.1	1.5 - 96.5	0.02
Group *conventional*	Group *Naturafarm*	4.8	1.3 - 18.3	0.02
Protofit plus Sprayfit	Whole milk plus Meliormilk	9.3	1.6 - 55.1	0.01

3.4. Risk factor analysis for abomasal lesions in the pyloric part

Management factors and animal breed showed no correlation ($p > 0.2$) with abomasal lesions in the pyloric part. In univariable logistic regression analysis, the type of feed, the cleaning intensity and carcass weight between 126 and 130 kg were weakly correlated ($0.05 < p < 0.2$) to abomasal lesions in the pyloric part (Table 6). A high correlation ($p < 0.05$) with an increased risk for pyloric lesions was observed for the ventilation type and a carcass weight above 130 kg. In multivariate logistic regression analysis, manual ventilation by windows was the only risk factor revealing a significant association with abomasal lesions in the pyloric part ($p = 0.035$, OR $=12.6$, 95% CI $=1.2–134.2$).

Table 6.
Factors associated (< 0.2) with the risk for occurrence of macroscopic pyloric lesions of veal calves at slaughter (univariable logistic regression)

Factor	Reference	Odds ratio	95% Confidence interval	Wald's p-value (p)
Amobolac + Gefumilk	Whole milk + Meliormilk	0.45	0.2 – 1.3	0.13
Cleaning the barn once per fattening period	Cleaning the barn more than once per fattening period	2.0	0.8 – 5.2	0.15
Carcass weight between 126 and 130 kg	Carcass weight less than 118 kg	2.5	- 0.2 – 2.1	0.12
Carcass weight above 130 kg	Carcass weight less than 118 kg	3.8	1.0 – 14.2	0.04
Manual ventilation by windows	Open fronted building	12.6	- 3.4 – 1.2	0.03

4. Discussion

In order to meet the consumers' expectations with respect to meat color, veal production in Switzerland involves the rearing of calves for 16 to 20 weeks mainly on milk or milk by-products. Thus, the final product is similar to white veal in Canada (Sargeant et al., 1994) or formula-fed veal in the USA (Schwartz, 1990). In Swiss settings, calves drink substantial amounts of liquid feed towards the end of the fattening period. Calves fed by bucket twice daily take up 10 liters per feeding session and calves fed ad libitum drink similar quantities. As opposed to the production of white veal and formula-fed veal, access to roughage is mandatory in Switzerland. As a rule, wheat straw is the only source of roughage for calves, but for particular settings meeting enhanced animal welfare standards on a voluntary basis. In these settings, calves are provided with hay. Whether feeding calves up to a body weight of 220 kg (carcass weight of 124 kg) with a liquid diet and with roughage of a high lignin content such as straw only is compatible with the calves' physiological needs and development of the forestomach system and abomasum remains questionable (Mattiello et al., 2002). In earlier studies, such a feeding regimen has been associated with an increased frequency of abomasal lesions (Ahmed et al., 2002; Groth and Berner, 1971). The goal of the present investigation, therefore, was to identify possible effects of two different production settings on the prevalence and distribution of abomasal lesions in veal calves. Over sixty calves from 'conventional' and 'Naturafarm' settings each were analyzed for fundic and pyloric lesions and findings were correlated with collected data on farm management. As the overall prevalence of abomasal lesions was above 25%, the number of animals studied allowed differences between settings to be assessed with a confidence level of 95% and a power of 80% (calculated with WinEpiscope 2.0, Epidecon, Wageningen University). Lesions were further categorized as Type 1 through 4 according to their severity. However, the number of animals examined was not sufficient to identify differences in the occurrence of single types of lesions.

Separate assessment of fundic and pyloric regions revealed a number of factors being involved in the development of abomasal lesions. Thus, univariable logistic regression analysis unveiled several factors being associated with an increased risk of fundic lesions. In order to account for factor levels and interactions between single factors, all risk factors with $p < 0.2$ were subjected to multivariate logistic regression analysis. This yielded the *feed type*, the *feeding technique* and the *conventional production setting* as such to be highly correlated with the occurrence of fundic lesions. As compared to the *'conventional'* settings, *'Naturafarm'* settings were characterized by a lower stocking density, the availability of an outside pen and by providing free access to water and hay. Although some aspects have not yet been resolved unequivocally, most of these factors have previously been considered to reduce chronic stress. Thus, the provision of water showed positive effects on non-nutritive oral behaviors and chronic stress indicators. Yet, no effect on the incidence of abomasal lesions was noted. In the respective study, however, the localization of lesions to different abomasal regions was ignored (Gottardo et al., 2002). Also, housing of young beef calves on pasture, i.e. at low stocking densities (Katchuik, 1992) decreased, and providing a coarse fiber source such as straw (Mattiello et al., 2002) increased the prevalence of abomasal lesions. On the other hand, Bokkers and Koene (2001) did not find any difference in the prevalence of abomasal lesions between three different housing systems. As these studies did not take into account the anatomical localization of the abomasal lesions, possible correlations may have been overlooked. This is consistent with the observation in the present study that the overall number of abomasal lesions did not correlate with the production setting. The notion that chronic stress increases the risk of fundic lesions is fully compatible with current pathogenetic concepts. Thus, a number of studies provide evidence that fundic and pyloric lesions result from different etiologies (Hemmingsen, 1966; Wensing et al., 1986). Dirksen (1994) and Pfeiffer (1992) reported that pathogenic mechanisms taking place in the fundic mucosa of the abomasum are similar to those leading to gastric ulcers in humans and other species. Thus, ulcerative processes in both cases are thought to result from the activation of the hypothalamo-pituitary-adrenal axis by chronic stress (Hessing et al., 1992; Katagiri et al., 2005; Lechin et al., 1994). 'Naturafarm' settings also differed from 'conventional' farms in terms of the feeding technique used. As for the observation that bucket feeding with an artificial teat (as practiced on 'conventional' farms only) increases the risk of fundic lesions as opposed to bucket feeding without teat, there is no ready explanation. It is known, however, that feeding twice daily is not enough to satisfy the calves' suckling needs, as calves kept with their mothers will suckle four up to ten times a day (de Passillé, 2001; Spinka and Illmann, 1992). As compared to the feeding of full milk together with Meliormilk, the combination of Protofit and Sprayfit turned out to be a risk factor for fundic lesions. Interestingly, the latter combination was used in both production settings. Therefore, this negative effect of feed composition must have been overruled by other management factors being specific to 'Naturafarm' settings. In other words, the prevalence of fundic lesions may be reduced even further when optimal feeding regimens are used under 'Naturafarm' conditions. The observation that a high percentage of vegetal ingredients such as soy protein, wheat starch and emulgators may elicit hypersensitivity reactions (Toullec and Lalles, 1996) with consecutive ulcerations provides a possible mechanism for the correlation observed. As the percentage of vegetal ingredients in Sprayfit unfortunately is not declared by the company, this hypothesis will need further investigations.

Seventy percent of all calves examined showed pyloric lesions. Yet, no difference in the prevalence of such lesions was noted between the production settings studied. This is compatible with a previously reported overall prevalence of 67% to 95% in studies not differentiating between different abomasal regions (Wiepkema et al., 1987; Groth and Berner, 1971). Notwithstanding, univariable logistic regression analysis disclosed a number of factors being associated with pyloric lesions. These included animal age and a high carcass weight (about 56% of body weight). In order to achieve a body weight of 240 kg on the basis of a liquid diet alone, daily feed uptake must increase steadily. Furthermore, group-housed calves compete for access to teats and are also displaced from teats while feeding (Jensen and Budde, 2006; von Keyserlingk *et al.*, 2004). Heavy animals are likely to be dominant individuals and, thus, to be able to take up large amounts of feed without being crowded out. These factors may lead to repeated gastric overload, distension and compression of the abomasal wall with consecutive hypoxic tissue damage to the mucosa especially in the funnel-shaped pyloric part (Krauser, 1987). Such a pathogenic mechanism is fully compatible with the observation that the prevalence of pyloric lesions does not differ between *ad libitum* feeding and bucket feeding twice daily. Thus, providing physiologically appropriate solid feed and slaughtering calves earlier (body weight about 180 kg) might reduce the prevalence of abomasal lesions in the pyloric part. When relevant single factors were subjected to multivariate logistic regression analysis, the only risk factor being closely associated with pyloric lesions was manual barn ventilation. As ventilation is unlikely to constitute a relevant factor in itself, the correlation may result from other factors being linked to manual ventilation but remaining unidentified in the present study.

In conclusion, requirements of high animal welfare such as low stocking density, access to an outside pen, the provision of hay and of water *ad libitum* reduce chronic stress situations and the prevalence of abomasal lesions in the fundic part. The beneficial effect of the *'Naturafarm'* production setting might be even further enhanced by optimizing the type of feed. In contrast, factors mentioned above do not affect the incidence of abomasal lesions in the pyloric part which are rather linked to the magnitude of milk intake per feeding session. In further investigations on abomasal lesions, it will be essential to take into account the anatomical localization of the lesions.

5. Acknowledgements

We thank the retailer 'Coop' for financing this research project, the personnel of the abattoir in Oensingen for their help in collecting the material and for providing carcass data, and the farmers for providing data on their farms. We also thank Dres. A. Ewy, Th. Kaufmann, A. Luginbühl, and D. Strabel for valuable discussions on calf health, husbandry, management and feeding practices, and Prof. Dr. F. Ehrensperger for debating on the histopathological results.

6. References

Ahmed, A. F., Constable, P. D., Misk, N. A., 2002. Effect of feeding frequency and route of administration on abomasal luminal pH in dairy calves fed milk replacer. Journal of Dairy Science **85**, 1502-8.

Bähler, C., 2007. Personal communication, unpublished.

Bokkers, E. A. M., Koene, P., 2001. Activity, oral behaviour and slaughter data as welfare indicators in veal calves: a comparison of three housing systems. Applied Animal Behaviour Science **75**, 1-75.

Braun, U., Eicher, R., Ehrensperger, F., 1991. Type 1 abomasal ulcers in dairy cattle. Zentralbl Veterinarmed A **38**, 357-66.

Cagalli, G. C., Bicego, C., Dall'Oea, A., Giuriolo, P., Menghini, E., 1995. Fattori amientali ed alimentari nelle patologie digestive del vitello "funzionalmente monogastrico", con particolare riferimento all'ucera abomasale, metodi die profilassi e terapia. Atti della Società Italiana di Buiatria **27**, 617-630.

Constable, P. D., Ahmed, A. F., Misk, N. A., 2005. Effect of suckling cow's milk or milk replacer on abomasal luminal pH in dairy calves. Journal of Veterinary Internal Medicine **19**, 97-102.

Coop, S., 2004. Coop's standards for Naturafarm.

de Passillé, A. M., 2001. Sucking motivation and related problems in calves. Appl Anim Behav Sci **72**, 175-187.

Dirksen, G., Doll, K., Einhellig, J., Seitz, A., Rademacher, G., Breitner, W., Klee, W., 1997. Labmagengeschwüre beim Kalb: klinische Untersuchungen und Erfahrungen. Tierärztliche Praxis **25**, 318-328.

Dirksen, G. U., 1994. Ulceration, dilatation and incarceration of the abomasum in calves: clinical investigations and experiences. The Bovine Practitioner **28**, 127-135.

Dyce, K. M., Sack, W. O., Wensing, C. J. G. (1991). "Anatomie der Haustiere," Ferdinand Enke Verlag.

Geishauser, T., 1989. Labmagengeschwür bei einem Kalb nach thermischer Enthornung ohne Betäubung. Tierärztliche Umschau **44**, 102-108.

Gesper, W., Dirksen, G., 1988. Experimentelle Untersuchungen über Diagnostik und Prophylaxe von Labmagengeschwüren beim Kalb. Inaugural-Dissertation.

Gottardo, F., Mattiello, S., Cozzi, G., Canali, E., Scanziani, E., Ravarotto, L., Ferrante, V., Verga, M., Andrighetto, I., 2002. The provision of drinking water to veal calves for welfare purposes. Journal of Animal Science **80**, 2362-72.

Groth, W., Berner, H., 1971. Comparative studies on the rumen content of fattening calves kept with and without litter and of early weaned calves. Deutsche Tierärztliche Wochenschrift **78**, 634-7 concl.

Hemmingsen, 1966. Erosiones et ulcera abomasi bovis. Nord. Vet.-Med. **18**, 354-365.

Hessing, M. J., Geudeke, M. J., Scheepens, C. J., Tielen, M. J., Schouten, W. G., Wiepkema, P. R., 1992. Mucosal lesions in the pars esophagus in swine: prevalence and the effect of stress. Tijdschr Diergeneeskd **117**, 445-50.

Jelinski, M. D., Ribble, C. S., Campbell, J. R., Janzen, E. D., 1996. Investigating the relationship between abomasal hairballs and perforating abomasal ulcers in unweaned beef calves. The Canadian Veterinary Journal **37**, 23-6.

Jensen, M. B., Budde, M., 2006. The effects of milk feeding method and group size on feeding behavior and cross-sucking in group-housed dairy calves. J Dairy Sci **89**, 4778-83.

Katagiri, F., Shiga, T., Sato, Y., Inoue, S., Itoh, H., Takeyama, M., 2005. Comparison of the effects of cytoprotective drugs on human plasma adrenocorticotropic hormone and cortisol levels with continual stress exposure. Biological & pharmaceutical bulletin **28**, 2146-8.

Katchuik, R., 1992. Abomasal disease in young beef calves: surgical findings and management factors. The Canadian Veterinary Journal **33**, 459-461.

Krauser, K., 1987. Pathogenesis of pyloric ulcers in the fattening calf. Berl Munch Tierarztl Wochenschr **100**, 156-61.

Lechin, F., van der Dijs, B., Lechin, A., Orozco, B., Lechin, M., Baez, S., Rada, I., Leon, G., Acosta, E., 1994. Plasma neurotransmitters and cortisol in chronic illness: role of stress. J Med **25**, 181-92.

Lensink, B. J., Fernandez, X., Boivin, X., Pradel, P., Le Neindre, P., Veissier, I., 2000. The impact of gentle contacts on ease of handling, welfare, and growth of calves and on quality of veal meat. Journal of Animal Science **78**, 1219-26.

Mattiello, S., Canali, E., Ferrante, V., Caniatti, M., Gottardo, F., Cozzi, G., Andrighetto, I., Verga, M., 2002. The provision of solid feeds to veal calves: II. Behavior, physiology, and abomasal damage. Journal of Animal Science **80**, 367-75.

Morisse, J. P., Huonnic, D., Cotte, J. P., Martrenchar, A., 2000. The effect of four fibrous feed supplementations on different welfare traits in veal calves. Animal Feed Science and Technology **84**, 129-136.

Navetat, H., 1987. Das Labmagengeschwür beim Kalb. Deutsche Tierärztliche Wochenschrift **94**, 282-4.

Pfeiffer, C. J., 1992. A review of spontaneous ulcer disease in domestic animals: chickens, cattle, horses, and swine. ACTA Physiologica Hungarica **80**, 149-58.

Prophet, E. B., Mills, B., Arrington, J. B., Sobin, L. H., 1994. Labaratory Methods in Histotechnology. American Registry of Pathology.

RAP (1999). "Fütterungsempfehlungen und Nährwerttabellen für Wiederkäuer," Zollikofen, Landwirtschaftliche Lehrmittelzentrale/Ed.

Sargeant, J. M., Blackwell, T. E., Martin, S. W., Tremblay, R. R., 1994. Production practices, calf health and mortality on six white veal farms in Ontario. Can J Vet Res **58**, 189-95.

Schwartz, A., 1990. The politics of formula-fed veal calf production. J Am Vet Med Assoc **196**, 1578-86.

Singh, G. B., Sharma, J. N., Kar, K., 1967. Pathogenesis of gastric ulceration produced under stress. J Path Bact **94**, 375-380.

Spinka, M., Illmann, G., 1992. Suckling behaviour of young dairy calves with their own and alien mother. Appl Anim Behav Sci **33**, 165-173.

Tierschutzgesetz 1978 www.admin.ch.

Toullec, R., Lalles, J. P., 1996. Verdauung von Proteinersatz-Futtermitteln bei Mastkälbern. AGRAR Forschung **3**, 427-430.

Veissier, I., Boissy, A., dePassille, A. M., Rushen, J., van Reenen, C. G., Roussel, S., Andanson, S., Pradel, P., 2001. Calves' responses to repeated social regrouping and relocation. Journal of Animal Science **79**, 2580-93.

von Keyserlingk, M. A., Brusius, L., Weary, D. M., 2004. Competition for teats and feeding behavior by group-housed dairy calves. J Dairy Sci **87**, 4190-4.

Welchman, D. D., Baust, G. N., 1987. A survey of abomasal ulceration in veal calves. The Veterinary Record **121**, 586-90.

Wensing, T., Breukink, H. J., van Dijk, S., 1986. The effect of feeding pellets of different types of roughage on the incidence of lesions in the abomasum of veal calves. Veterinary Research Communications **10**, 195-202.

Wiepkema, P. R., Van Hellemond, K. K., Roessingh, P., Romberg, H., 1987. Behaviour and abomasal damage in individual veal calves. Applied Animal Behaviour Science **18**, 257-268.

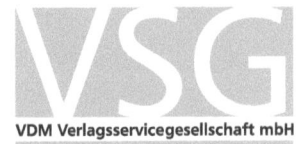

Die VDM Verlagsservicegesellschaft sucht für wissenschaftliche Verlage abgeschlossene und herausragende

Dissertationen, Habilitationen, Diplomarbeiten, Master Theses, Magisterarbeiten usw.

für die kostenlose Publikation als Fachbuch.

Sie verfügen über eine Arbeit, die hohen inhaltlichen und formalen Ansprüchen genügt, und haben Interesse an einer honorarvergüteten Publikation?

Dann senden Sie bitte erste Informationen über sich und Ihre Arbeit per Email an *info@vdm-vsg.de*.

Sie erhalten kurzfristig unser Feedback!

VDM Verlagsservicegesellschaft mbH
Dudweiler Landstr. 99   Telefon +49 681 3720 174
D - 66123 Saarbrücken   Fax   +49 681 3720 1749

www.vdm-vsg.de

Die VDM Verlagsservicegesellschaft mbH vertritt

 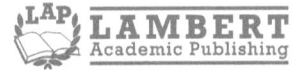 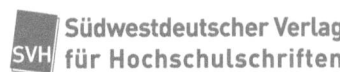

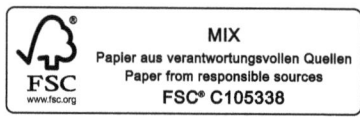

Printed by Books on Demand GmbH, Norderstedt / Germany